DISCOVER THE MEDITERRANEAN DIET

A Delicious Path to Health and Longevity

Dr. Raymond F. Bernard

TABLE OF CONTENTS

CHAPTER 1

Mediterranean Diet

Welcome to the enchanting world of the Mediterranean diet, a culinary journey that will not only tantalize your taste buds but also nourish your body and soul. In this chapter, we embark on an exploration of this time-honored eating pattern, delving into its history, cultural significance, the plethora of health benefits it offers, and an overview of what you can expect to discover in the rest of this book.

The Mediterranean Diet: A Culinary Tradition

The Mediterranean diet is far more than just a list of foods; it's a way of life that has been practiced for centuries in the regions bordering the Mediterranean Sea, including Greece, Southern Italy, Spain, and parts of North Africa and the Middle East. At its core, this diet reflects the eating habits of these communities, and it's deeply intertwined with their culture, traditions, and lifestyle.

A Brief Glimpse into History

To truly understand the essence of the Mediterranean diet, we must journey back in time. Its origins can be traced to ancient civilizations such as the Greeks and the Romans. These societies revered the Mediterranean as the cradle of their culinary wisdom, believing that their diet not only sustained their bodies but also nurtured their minds and spirits.

The diet was largely born out of necessity. People living around the Mediterranean had access to an abundance of fruits, vegetables, grains, olive oil, and seafood. These staples formed the foundation of their diet out of sheer practicality, and over time, this diet has proven to be one of the healthiest in the world.

Cultural Significance

The Mediterranean diet isn't just about the food you eat; it's also about the way you eat it. Family gatherings around the dinner table are a sacred tradition in Mediterranean cultures. These meals are occasions for bonding, storytelling, and laughter, and they often extend for hours. Meals are savored, not rushed, and there's a profound sense of appreciation for the flavors and textures of each dish.

Community and social connections are fundamental aspects of Mediterranean life. The act of sharing a meal is seen as an expression of love and friendship. It's a moment to connect with loved ones, fostering a sense of belonging and well-being.

Health Benefits: Science-Backed Wellness

One of the key reasons the Mediterranean diet has captured global attention is its impressive array of health benefits. Research consistently shows that people who follow this dietary pattern are less prone to a variety of chronic diseases and tend to live longer, healthier lives. Here's a glimpse of what you can expect:

- **Heart Health**: A cornerstone of the Mediterranean diet is olive oil, which is rich in monounsaturated fats. These fats are known to lower bad cholesterol levels, reducing the risk of heart disease. Additionally, the diet's emphasis on fruits, vegetables, and whole grains provides a wealth of antioxidants, fiber, and nutrients that support cardiovascular health.

- **Weight Management**: While not a strict "weight-loss" diet, the Mediterranean way of eating naturally promotes a healthy weight. The focus on whole, unprocessed foods, along with the inclusion of healthy fats, helps control appetite and prevent overeating.

- **Diabetes Management**: Studies have shown that the Mediterranean diet can help manage and even prevent type 2 diabetes. Its high-fiber content and low glycemic index foods help regulate blood sugar levels.

- **Brain Health**: The Mediterranean diet's abundance of antioxidants, omega-3 fatty acids from fish, and other nutrients has been linked to improved cognitive function and a reduced risk of age-related cognitive decline.

- **Cancer Prevention**: Some components of the Mediterranean diet, such as the phytonutrients in fruits and vegetables and the protective effects of olive oil, have been associated with a lower risk of certain types of cancer.

- **Longevity**: People living in Mediterranean regions have some of the highest life expectancies in the world, and much of this can be attributed to their diet and lifestyle.

What to Expect in This Book

Now that you've glimpsed the tantalizing allure of the Mediterranean diet, let's discuss what you can expect to find in the upcoming chapters of this book.

We've structured this book to be both informative and practical, ensuring that you not only understand the principles of the diet but also have the tools and knowledge to incorporate it into your own life.

In the following chapters:

- **Chapter 2: The Mediterranean Way of Life** delves deeper into the lifestyle aspects of this diet, exploring how the Mediterranean way of life contributes to overall well-being.

- **Chapter 3: The Mediterranean Diet Pyramid** breaks down the dietary framework, giving you a visual representation of the foods you should prioritize and those you should enjoy in moderation.

- **Chapters 4 through 9** will explore the key food groups that form the foundation of the Mediterranean diet. We'll dive into fruits and vegetables, grains and legumes, olive oil and healthy fats, lean proteins, dairy and dairy alternatives, and the rich world of

Mediterranean herbs, spices, and flavors. For each of these food groups, we'll provide insights into their role in the diet, their health benefits, and a treasure trove of delicious recipes.

- **Chapter 10: Putting It All Together** brings everything full circle. It offers practical guidance on how to create your own Mediterranean meal plan, providing tips and suggestions to help you succeed on your culinary journey. You'll also find success stories and testimonials from individuals who have experienced the transformational power of the Mediterranean diet.

In the appendix, we've included valuable resources such as Mediterranean diet meal plans, grocery shopping lists, conversion charts, and a glossary of Mediterranean ingredients to assist you on your journey.

So, whether you're looking to improve your health, savor exquisite flavors, or simply explore a new way of eating, this book will be your trusted companion. The Mediterranean diet is not a fad;

it's a timeless and proven path to wellness and culinary delight. So, let's embark on this journey together, and may it bring you health, happiness, and a newfound appreciation for the art of Mediterranean living.

CHAPTER 2

The Mediterranean Way of Life

In the previous chapter, we introduced you to the essence of the Mediterranean diet – a delicious and nutritious way of eating rooted in centuries-old traditions. Now, let's delve deeper into the heart of the Mediterranean lifestyle and understand why it's not just about what you eat, but how you live.

A Culture of Connection

At the core of the Mediterranean way of life is a deep sense of community and connection. The dinner table is not just a place to refuel but a place to reconnect with loved ones. Meals are a social event, a daily ritual where families and friends gather, share stories, and forge bonds. The act of dining together is seen as an expression of love and togetherness.

In contrast to the hurried pace of modern life, Mediterranean meals are unhurried affairs, often stretching for hours. This leisurely approach to eating allows for the full appreciation of flavors and textures, promoting mindfulness and reducing the tendency to overeat. In this chapter, we explore the cultural significance of these communal meals and how they contribute to a sense of well-being.

The Role of Family and Community

The Mediterranean way of life places a high value on family and community. Meals are occasions for bringing people together, reinforcing bonds, and fostering a sense of belonging. Whether it's a bustling family dinner or a festive community celebration, the

Mediterranean culture thrives on shared culinary experiences.

This emphasis on social connection has profound implications for mental and emotional health. Research shows that strong social ties are associated with lower rates of depression and increased life satisfaction. In the Mediterranean, the act of gathering around the table serves as a powerful antidote to the isolation that can plague our fast-paced, digitally-driven lives.

Leisure and Enjoyment

In Mediterranean cultures, there's an emphasis on enjoying life to the fullest. The idea of "la dolce vita" – the sweet life – is not just a catchphrase but a philosophy. Leisure activities, such as strolling through picturesque villages, sipping espresso at a café, or lounging on a sun-drenched beach, are valued and prioritized.

This leisurely approach to life extends to mealtime as well. Unlike rushed office lunches or eating on the go, Mediterranean meals are an invitation to slow down, savor each bite, and engage in lively conversations. This approach to dining is not only more pleasurable but also healthier, as it allows the body to recognize satiety cues and prevent overeating.

Nature's Rhythms and Seasonal Eating

Mediterranean communities have a deep respect for the natural rhythms of the seasons. Their diets are influenced by the availability of fresh, locally grown produce. This concept of seasonal eating not only ensures that meals are packed with flavor and nutrients but also promotes sustainability.

In the spring, there's an abundance of tender greens, asparagus, and artichokes. Summer brings an explosion of tomatoes, cucumbers, and peppers. Autumn ushers in a harvest of figs, grapes, and olives. And in winter, hearty greens, citrus fruits, and root vegetables take center stage. This reliance on seasonal ingredients not only keeps meals exciting and diverse but also aligns with the principles of sustainable and environmentally friendly eating.

Physical Activity and Mediterranean Living

Physical activity is woven into the fabric of Mediterranean living. In many Mediterranean communities, walking is the primary mode of transportation. People stroll through their neighborhoods, visit local markets, and engage in outdoor activities as a part of their daily routine.

This natural, integrated approach to physical activity promotes health and vitality. Walking is not seen as a chore but as a joyful way to connect with the environment and one's community. The Mediterranean lifestyle encourages people to enjoy the outdoors, whether it's a hike in the hills, a swim in the sea, or a leisurely bike ride through scenic countryside.

Stress Reduction and Mediterranean Mindfulness

In today's fast-paced world, stress is a common companion. However, Mediterranean living offers strategies to manage and reduce stress. The combination of leisurely meals, strong social connections, physical activity, and a focus on relaxation contributes to lower stress levels in these cultures.

Mediterranean mindfulness is about being fully present in the moment, whether you're savoring a forkful of roasted vegetables, sharing a laugh with a friend, or watching the sunset over the sea. This mindfulness practice can be a powerful antidote to the anxiety and stress that often accompany modern life.

A Blueprint for Well-Being

In summary, the Mediterranean way of life is more than a mere dietary plan; it's a holistic approach to well-being. It recognizes that what you eat is just one part of the equation, and equally important is how you live. The emphasis on family, community, leisure, seasonal eating, physical activity, and mindfulness all contribute to a higher quality of life.

As we journey through the chapters of this book, we'll continue to explore the practical aspects of the Mediterranean diet, from the foods you should include in your meals to delicious recipes that will transport you to the shores of the Mediterranean. However, never forget that adopting the Mediterranean way of life isn't just about what's on your plate; it's about embracing a philosophy that celebrates the art of living well.

So, as you dive into this culinary adventure, keep in mind the cultural and lifestyle elements that make the Mediterranean diet a truly holistic approach to health and happiness. Embrace the traditions, savor the flavors, and relish the joy of the Mediterranean way of life. In doing so, you'll not only nourish your body but also nurture your spirit and enrich your life in countless ways.

CHAPTER 3

The Mediterranean Diet Pyramid

In this chapter, we will take a closer look at the iconic symbol of the Mediterranean diet - the Mediterranean Diet Pyramid. This pyramid serves as a visual representation of the dietary framework that has been at the heart of the Mediterranean way of eating for generations. By understanding its layers and principles, you'll gain valuable insights into how to structure your meals for both health and culinary pleasure.

Foundation: Plant-Based Foods

The foundation of the Mediterranean Diet Pyramid is a lush and diverse assortment of plant-based foods. These foods form the bedrock of the diet and are consumed in abundance. Here's a breakdown of the essential components in this category:

- **Fruits and Vegetables**: Fruits and vegetables are the shining stars of the

Mediterranean diet. Rich in vitamins, minerals, fiber, and antioxidants, they are a powerhouse of nutrition. The Mediterranean tradition encourages the consumption of a wide variety of colorful produce, such as tomatoes, peppers, eggplants, spinach, and citrus fruits.

- **Whole Grains**: Whole grains, such as whole wheat bread, pasta, and couscous, are favored over refined grains. They provide sustained energy, fiber, and a host of essential nutrients.

- **Legumes**: Beans, lentils, and chickpeas are staples in Mediterranean cuisine. They are not only a source of plant-based protein but also fiber and various vitamins and minerals.

Middle Layer: Healthy Fats

One of the most distinctive features of the Mediterranean diet is its use of healthy fats as a primary source of dietary energy. Olive oil, in particular, takes center stage in this category, and it's used generously in cooking and as a dressing for salads. Here's a closer look at the fats found in this layer:

- **Olive Oil**: Extra virgin olive oil is rich in monounsaturated fats, particularly oleic acid, which is associated with various health benefits, including heart health. It's a key source of flavor and healthy fats in Mediterranean dishes.

- **Nuts and Seeds**: Almonds, walnuts, and other nuts and seeds are included for their healthy fats, protein, and fiber. They make great snacks and can be sprinkled on salads and added to dishes for extra crunch and flavor.

Protein Sources

The next layer of the Mediterranean Diet Pyramid is dedicated to protein sources, which include both animal and plant-based options. This flexibility allows individuals to adapt the diet to their preferences and dietary restrictions. Here are the primary protein sources:

- **Fish and Seafood**: Fish, particularly fatty fish like

salmon, mackerel, and sardines, are featured prominently. They provide omega-3 fatty acids, which are known for their heart-protective benefits. Grilled or baked fish is a staple in Mediterranean cuisine.

- **Poultry**: Chicken and turkey are included but are typically consumed in smaller quantities than fish. They are often prepared with flavorful herbs and spices.

- **Legumes and Nuts**: As mentioned earlier, legumes like beans and lentils, as well as nuts and seeds, provide plant-based protein. They are used in a wide range of Mediterranean dishes, from hummus to bean salads.

- **Dairy**: While dairy is not a primary protein source, it's included in moderation. Yogurt and cheese, especially varieties like feta and Greek yogurt, are common in Mediterranean meals.

Occasional Foods

At the top of the Mediterranean Diet Pyramid are foods that should be consumed only occasionally. These include:

- **Sweets and Desserts**: Traditional Mediterranean desserts tend to be less sweet and indulgent than those found in many Western cultures. They may include items like baklava, honey-drizzled pastries, or fresh fruit.

- **Red Meat**: Red meat, such as beef and lamb, is eaten less frequently in Mediterranean diets compared to other protein sources. When consumed, it's often in smaller portions and as part of a larger dish, such as in a kebab or stew.

- **Processed Foods**: Highly processed foods and sugary beverages are discouraged in the Mediterranean diet. The focus is on whole, natural foods.

Moderate Consumption of Wine

A notable feature of the Mediterranean Diet Pyramid is the inclusion of wine, particularly red wine, in moderation. Many Mediterranean cultures enjoy a glass of wine with meals. The antioxidants and potential heart benefits of red wine have been studied and are often cited as part of the Mediterranean diet's healthful qualities. However, it's essential to emphasize moderation – excessive alcohol consumption can have adverse health effects.

Fluids and Hydration

In addition to wine, water is a fundamental component of the Mediterranean diet. Staying well-hydrated is crucial for overall health. Herbal teas, such as chamomile and mint, are also popular and complement the Mediterranean flavor profile.

Putting It All Together

Understanding the Mediterranean Diet Pyramid provides a clear blueprint for structuring your meals. At the base, you have a generous array of fruits, vegetables, whole grains, and legumes. These should make up a significant portion of your daily intake, providing essential vitamins, minerals, and fiber.

The middle layer introduces healthy fats, particularly olive oil and nuts, which should be incorporated into your meals for flavor and nutritional benefits.

For protein, you have choices that suit various dietary preferences, from fish and seafood to poultry, legumes, and dairy. These sources offer protein, essential fats, and other vital nutrients.

Occasional indulgences like sweets, red meat, and processed foods should be enjoyed sparingly, with a focus on moderation.

The Mediterranean diet's emphasis on balanced and varied eating not only promotes health but also culinary satisfaction. It's a way of eating that allows for creativity and exploration in the kitchen while delivering a wealth of nutrients and flavors.

Customizing Your Mediterranean Plate

The Mediterranean Diet Pyramid provides a strong foundation, but it's also flexible. You can adapt it to your individual dietary needs, preferences, and cultural traditions. Whether you're vegetarian, pescatarian, or have specific dietary requirements, the Mediterranean diet offers room for customization.

In the chapters that follow, we'll explore each of these layers in more detail, providing you with a wealth of information, tips, and delicious recipes that will inspire you to create Mediterranean-inspired dishes that suit your tastes and lifestyle.

By embracing the principles of the Mediterranean Diet Pyramid, you'll not only enjoy the culinary delights of this ancient way of eating but also reap the numerous health benefits it offers. So, let's embark on this gastronomic journey together, as we explore the vibrant flavors and nourishing traditions of the Mediterranean diet.

CHAPTER 4

Fruits and Vegetables

In this chapter, we delve into the vibrant world of fruits and vegetables, the cornerstone of the Mediterranean diet. These colorful and nutritious treasures are not just ingredients; they are the essence of Mediterranean cuisine. Here, we'll explore the vital role they play in the diet, their seasonal significance, and offer a taste of the delicious Mediterranean recipes that highlight these essential ingredients.

A Rainbow of Nutrients

Fruits and vegetables are celebrated in Mediterranean cuisine for their exceptional nutritional value. They are packed with vitamins, minerals, fiber, and antioxidants, all of which contribute to good health and well-being. The Mediterranean diet encourages a diverse and colorful array of produce, providing a wide range of nutrients.

- **Vitamins and Minerals**: Fruits and vegetables are rich in essential vitamins like vitamin C, vitamin A, and various B vitamins. They are also abundant sources of minerals like potassium, magnesium, and folate, which are vital for various bodily functions.

- **Antioxidants**: Many fruits and vegetables are loaded with antioxidants, such as flavonoids and carotenoids, which help protect cells from oxidative damage and reduce the risk of chronic diseases.

- **Fiber**: The fiber content in these foods supports digestive health, helps maintain a healthy weight, and aids in regulating blood sugar levels.

Seasonal Eating and Local Produce

A fundamental aspect of Mediterranean eating is seasonal and locally sourced ingredients. This approach aligns with the natural rhythms of the earth, ensuring that you enjoy produce at its peak flavor and nutritional value. It's a practice that connects people with their environment and promotes sustainability.

In spring, you'll savor tender asparagus, artichokes, and

strawberries. Summer brings the juicy sweetness of tomatoes, cucumbers, and watermelon. Autumn introduces figs, grapes, and pomegranates, while winter offers hearty greens, citrus fruits, and root vegetables. Seasonal eating ensures that your meals are always fresh, flavorful, and in harmony with the changing seasons.

Mediterranean Fruit and Vegetable Staples

1. **Tomatoes**: Tomatoes are a Mediterranean superstar, often used in salads, sauces, and soups. They're not only

delicious but also a rich source of the antioxidant lycopene, known for its potential role in reducing the risk of certain cancers.

2. **Olives**: Olives and olive products are ubiquitous in Mediterranean cuisine. They provide healthy fats and a unique flavor profile. Olives can be enjoyed as a snack or used to garnish dishes, while olive oil is the go-to cooking fat and salad dressing.

3. **Eggplants**: Eggplants, or aubergines, are versatile vegetables used in dishes like moussaka and caponata.

They are a good source of dietary fiber and antioxidants.

4. **Zucchini and Squash**: These summer vegetables are abundant in Mediterranean gardens. They can be sautéed, grilled, or stuffed, and they add a delightful mild flavor to many dishes.

5. **Citrus Fruits**: Oranges, lemons, and grapefruits are abundant in Mediterranean regions. They add zesty brightness to salads, desserts, and marinades,

and are a rich source of vitamin C.

6. **Leafy Greens**: Mediterranean cuisines make good use of leafy greens like spinach, Swiss chard, and arugula. They are rich in vitamins and minerals, especially iron and calcium.

Cooking Techniques for Maximum Flavor

Mediterranean cooking showcases the natural flavors of fruits and vegetables through various cooking techniques. Here are a few methods commonly used:

- **Grilling**: Vegetables like eggplant, zucchini, and bell peppers are often grilled, enhancing their smoky flavors.

- **Roasting**: Roasting tomatoes, peppers, and root vegetables concentrates their sweetness and adds depth to dishes.

- **Sautéing**: Quick sautés with olive oil and garlic are a common way to prepare leafy greens and other vegetables.

- **Steaming**: Steaming vegetables preserves their color and nutrients. It's often used for greens and delicate vegetables.

- **Raw**: Many Mediterranean salads feature raw vegetables, allowing their natural crunch and freshness to shine through.

Mediterranean Recipes Showcasing Fruits and Vegetables

Now, let's indulge in a taste of the Mediterranean with some mouthwatering recipes:

1. **Greek Salad**: A classic Greek salad is a vibrant combination of tomatoes,

cucumbers, bell peppers, red onions, olives, and feta cheese, all drizzled with olive oil and sprinkled with oregano. It's a refreshing and nutrient-packed dish.

2. **Ratatouille**: This Provençal vegetable medley features eggplant, zucchini, bell peppers, and tomatoes, all simmered in olive oil and herbs until tender. It's a delightful taste of summer.

3. **Caprese Salad**: A simple Italian favorite, Caprese salad combines ripe tomatoes, fresh mozzarella cheese, and basil leaves,

drizzled with olive oil and balsamic vinegar. It's a celebration of seasonal ingredients.

4. **Tzatziki**: This creamy Greek dip is made from yogurt, cucumbers, garlic, and fresh dill. It's a refreshing accompaniment to grilled vegetables or pita bread.

5. **Roasted Red Pepper Hummus**: This Mediterranean twist on hummus incorporates roasted red peppers for a smoky, sweet flavor. It's

perfect for dipping fresh vegetables or pita bread.

The Mediterranean Approach: Health and Pleasure

Beyond their nutritional value, fruits and vegetables are central to the Mediterranean diet because they embody the core principles of this way of eating – health and pleasure. They nourish the body with essential nutrients while delighting the senses with their colors, flavors, and textures.

In Mediterranean cultures, meals are not just about sustenance; they are a celebration of life, a moment to savor the beauty of the natural world, and an opportunity to connect with loved ones. As you explore the Mediterranean diet, remember that it's not about deprivation or strict rules; it's about embracing a way of eating that brings joy and fulfillment to your daily life.

So, whether you're savoring the crisp bite of a Mediterranean salad or relishing the rich flavors of a roasted vegetable dish, you're not just nourishing your body – you're celebrating the profound connection between food, health, and the sheer pleasure of the culinary experience. In the chapters that follow, we'll continue to explore the delicious and healthful elements of the Mediterranean diet, guiding you toward a deeper understanding and appreciation of this remarkable way of eating.

CHAPTER 5

Grains and Legumes

In the vibrant mosaic of the Mediterranean diet, grains and legumes form a hearty and wholesome foundation. These humble yet nutritious staples have been cherished for centuries in Mediterranean cultures, and in this chapter, we'll delve into their essential role, the health benefits they offer, and we'll tantalize your taste buds with some classic Mediterranean recipes.

The Mediterranean Love Affair with Grains and Legumes

Grains and legumes are the workhorses of Mediterranean cuisine. They provide sustenance, fiber, and a wealth of essential nutrients. Here's a closer look at why they hold such a cherished place in this dietary tradition:

1. Grains: The Staff of Life

Whole Grains: The Mediterranean diet places a strong emphasis on whole grains, such as whole wheat, oats, barley, and brown rice. Unlike refined grains, whole grains retain the bran and germ, which are rich in fiber, vitamins, minerals, and antioxidants. This makes them a more nutritious choice and an excellent source of sustained energy.

Bread: Bread is a fundamental part of Mediterranean meals. Traditional artisanal bread, like Italian ciabatta or French baguette, is often made with simple ingredients: flour, water, yeast, and salt. It's enjoyed with olive oil, used as a base for bruschetta, or as a side to soak up sauces and juices in various dishes.

Pasta: Pasta is an Italian gift to the culinary world, and it's a staple in the Mediterranean diet. Whole-grain pasta varieties offer the same comforting experience with an added nutritional boost.

2. Legumes: Plant-Based Protein Powerhouses

Beans: Beans come in a variety of forms in Mediterranean cuisine, from chickpeas (garbanzo beans) to lentils, kidney beans, and cannellini beans. They are versatile, affordable, and rich in protein, fiber, and essential minerals.

Lentils: Lentils are particularly cherished for their quick cooking time and high nutritional value. They are featured in soups, salads, and stews throughout the Mediterranean region.

Hummus: Hummus, a creamy dip made from pureed chickpeas, tahini (sesame seed paste), lemon juice, and garlic, is a beloved staple. It's a delightful snack, sandwich spread, or appetizer.

Health Benefits of Grains and Legumes

The inclusion of grains and legumes in the Mediterranean diet contributes significantly to its numerous health benefits:

1. **Heart Health**: The fiber in whole grains and legumes helps lower cholesterol levels and reduce the risk of heart disease. They also provide potassium, which supports healthy blood pressure.

2. **Weight Management**: The fiber and protein in these staples promote a feeling of fullness and satisfaction, reducing the likelihood of overeating and aiding in weight management.

3. Blood Sugar Control: The slow-release carbohydrates in whole grains and legumes help regulate blood sugar levels, making them suitable choices for individuals with diabetes or those looking to prevent it.

4. Digestive Health: The fiber content aids in regular bowel movements and supports a healthy digestive system.

5. Nutrient Density: Grains and legumes are nutrient-dense foods, meaning they provide a significant amount of vitamins, minerals, and antioxidants relative to their calorie content.

6. Plant-Based Protein: For those following a vegetarian or vegan diet, legumes are an excellent source of plant-based protein, helping meet protein needs without animal products.

Delicious Mediterranean Dishes: Recipes to Savor

Now, let's tantalize your taste buds with some classic Mediterranean recipes that feature grains and legumes:

1. Risotto: This creamy Italian rice dish is a canvas for creativity. Try a classic mushroom risotto

with Arborio rice or experiment
with whole-grain variations.

2. Minestrone Soup:
Minestrone is a hearty Italian
vegetable soup that often includes
beans, pasta, and a rich tomato
broth.

3. Mujadara: A Middle Eastern
dish made with lentils, rice, and
caramelized onions, Mujadara is a
simple yet flavorful dish often
garnished with yogurt and fresh
herbs.

4. Greek Chickpea Salad: A
fresh and zesty salad featuring
chickpeas, cucumber, tomatoes,

olives, and feta cheese, all drizzled with olive oil and lemon juice.

5. Tabbouleh: A vibrant Middle Eastern salad made with bulgur wheat, fresh parsley, mint, tomatoes, and a lemony dressing.

6. Pasta e Fagioli: An Italian pasta and bean soup, hearty with whole-grain pasta, beans, and a rich tomato-based broth.

Balancing Grains and Legumes in Your Diet

Incorporating grains and legumes into your Mediterranean-inspired meals is both nutritious and delicious. Here are some tips for balancing these staples in your diet:

1. Diversify Your Choices: Experiment with different grains like quinoa, farro, or freekeh. Likewise, explore various legumes beyond the usual suspects, such as black-eyed peas, butter beans, or mung beans.

2. Portion Control: While these foods are nutritious, portion control is key. Keep serving sizes reasonable, and balance them with plenty of vegetables and lean proteins.

3. Whole Grains vs. Refined Grains: Whenever possible, opt for whole grains over refined grains like white rice or white bread. Whole grains offer more fiber and nutrients.

4. Legume Varieties: Choose legumes in a range of colors, sizes, and shapes. Each type has its unique flavor and texture, adding diversity to your meals.

5. Bean Soups and Stews: Create hearty soups and stews by combining legumes with vegetables and lean proteins. These dishes are not only satisfying but also perfect for batch cooking.

6. Pasta Pairings: When enjoying pasta, balance it with plenty of vegetables, lean proteins, and a flavorful sauce made from fresh ingredients and olive oil.

Customizing for Dietary Preferences

The Mediterranean diet is versatile and adaptable, making it suitable for various dietary preferences and restrictions. Whether you're vegetarian, vegan, gluten-free, or have specific dietary requirements, grains and legumes offer flexibility.

Vegetarian and Vegan Diets: Grains and legumes provide essential protein and nutrients for those following plant-based diets. Incorporate them into a variety of dishes for balanced nutrition.

Gluten-Free: If you're gluten-free, explore naturally gluten-free grains like rice, quinoa, and cornmeal. Ensure that legumes are not cross-contaminated with gluten during processing.

Balancing Act: For those with specific dietary requirements, consider working with a registered dietitian or nutritionist to create a balanced Mediterranean diet plan that meets your individual needs.

In Conclusion

Grains and legumes are the unsung heroes of the Mediterranean diet, offering a bounty of health benefits and culinary delight. As you explore these staples in your culinary journey, remember that the Mediterranean way of eating is not just about nourishing your body but also celebrating the traditions and flavors that have stood the test of time.

In the chapters that follow, we'll continue to unearth the treasures of the Mediterranean diet, from the heart-healthy fats of olive oil to the succulent proteins of seafood. Each component adds to the rich tapestry of flavors and nutrition that make this diet a true embodiment of health and pleasure. So, savor the wholesome goodness of grains and legumes, and let them be a reminder that in Mediterranean cuisine, even the simplest ingredients can create culinary magic.

CHAPTER 6

Olive Oil and Healthy Fats

In the enchanting realm of Mediterranean cuisine, olive oil takes center stage as the golden elixir of life. In this chapter, we'll dive deep into the Mediterranean's love affair with olive oil and explore the world of healthy fats. We'll uncover why olive oil is cherished, its myriad health benefits, and how it fits into the broader landscape of fats in the Mediterranean diet.

Olive Oil: Liquid Gold of the Mediterranean

Olive oil, often referred to as "liquid gold," is the backbone of Mediterranean cooking. It's not just a cooking ingredient; it's a symbol of life, health, and prosperity. Here's why olive oil is so highly esteemed:

1. History and Tradition: The cultivation of olive trees and the production of olive oil have been central to Mediterranean culture for millennia. This rich history has imbued olive oil with deep cultural significance.

2. Versatility: Olive oil is remarkably versatile. It serves as a cooking medium, a salad dressing, a dip for bread, and even a flavor enhancer for countless dishes. Its mild, fruity flavor complements a wide range of ingredients.

3. Nutrient-Rich: Olive oil is a nutritional powerhouse. It's predominantly composed of monounsaturated fats, primarily oleic acid, which is associated with numerous health benefits. It's also rich in antioxidants, vitamin E, and anti-inflammatory compounds.

4.   Heart-Healthy: The monounsaturated fats in olive oil have been extensively studied for their role in promoting heart health. Regular consumption has been linked to reduced risk factors for heart disease, including lower LDL (bad) cholesterol levels.

5.   Antioxidant   Properties: Olive oil contains antioxidants like polyphenols, which help protect cells from oxidative damage and inflammation, potentially reducing the risk of chronic diseases.

6. Anti-Inflammatory Effects: Some of the compounds in olive oil have been shown to have anti-inflammatory properties, which are believed to contribute to its health benefits.

7. Culinary Delight: Beyond its health attributes, olive oil is simply delicious. Its unique flavor enhances a wide range of dishes, from drizzling over fresh vegetables to infusing the rich flavor of a pasta sauce.

Categories of Olive Oil

Not all olive oils are created equal. The Mediterranean region offers a wide range of olive oil varieties, each with its own flavor profile and culinary use. Here are the main categories:

1. Extra Virgin Olive Oil: This is the highest quality olive oil, obtained from the first cold pressing of the olives. It has a rich, fruity flavor and is often used for dressings, dips, and finishing dishes.

2. Virgin Olive Oil: Slightly lower in quality than extra virgin, virgin olive oil is also obtained from the first pressing of olives. It has a milder flavor and can be used in similar ways to extra virgin.

3. Pure Olive Oil: Sometimes labeled simply as "olive oil," this type is a blend of virgin and refined olive oils. It has a neutral flavor and is suitable for cooking, especially at higher temperatures.

4. Olive Pomace Oil: This oil is extracted from the pulp and pits of olives after the initial pressing. It's the least expensive and has a mild, neutral flavor. It's often used for frying and cooking at high temperatures.

Health Benefits of Olive Oil and Healthy Fats

Olive oil, along with other healthy fats found in the Mediterranean diet, plays a vital role in promoting overall well-being. Here's a look at the health benefits of incorporating these fats into your diet:

1. **Heart Health**: The monounsaturated fats in olive oil are known to lower LDL (bad) cholesterol levels, reducing the risk of heart disease. They also help maintain healthy blood vessel function.

2. **Weight Management**: Olive oil's healthy fats help control appetite and promote feelings of

fullness, aiding in weight management.

3. Anti-Inflammatory Effects: Some components of olive oil, particularly the polyphenols, exhibit anti-inflammatory properties, which may help protect against chronic diseases.

4. Cognitive Health: Olive oil's antioxidants and monounsaturated fats have been linked to improved cognitive function and a reduced risk of age-related cognitive decline.

5. Diabetes Management: The Mediterranean diet, which

includes olive oil, has been shown to help manage blood sugar levels in individuals with diabetes.

6. Skin Health: The antioxidants in olive oil can help protect the skin from damage caused by free radicals and UV rays. Olive oil is also a natural moisturizer.

7. Digestive Health: The monounsaturated fats in olive oil can support healthy digestion and may help reduce the risk of digestive disorders.

Balancing Healthy Fats in the Mediterranean Diet

While olive oil is a superstar in the Mediterranean diet, it's not the only source of healthy fats. A well-rounded Mediterranean diet includes a variety of fats to provide a balanced and enjoyable culinary experience. Here's how you can balance healthy fats in your diet:

1. **Olive Oil**: Make extra virgin olive oil your primary cooking fat and salad dressing. Its distinct flavor adds depth to dishes.

2. **Nuts and Seeds**: Incorporate a variety of nuts and seeds into your diet. Almonds, walnuts, flaxseeds, and chia seeds are excellent choices.

3. Fatty Fish: Enjoy fatty fish like salmon, mackerel, and sardines at least twice a week. They are rich in omega-3 fatty acids, which are highly beneficial for heart and brain health.

4. Avocado: Avocado is another Mediterranean favorite. Its creamy texture and healthy fats make it a versatile ingredient for salads, sandwiches, and dips like guacamole.

5. Dairy: If you consume dairy, choose low-fat or Greek yogurt for added protein and healthy fats.

6. Balanced Cooking: While olive oil is ideal for low to medium heat cooking, use other fats like canola oil or grapeseed oil for high-heat cooking.

Customizing for Dietary Preferences

The Mediterranean diet is flexible and can be adapted to various dietary preferences:

Vegetarian and Vegan Diets: Olive oil and plant-based fats are integral to vegetarian and vegan Mediterranean diets. You'll find ample options for creating flavorful and nutritious meals.

Low-Fat Diets: For those following a low-fat diet, focus on minimizing added fats and oils. Use olive oil sparingly and emphasize lean proteins and whole grains.

Balanced Approach: For most individuals, a balanced approach that includes a variety of healthy fats, including olive oil, nuts, seeds, and fatty fish, offers the best combination of flavor and nutrition.

In Conclusion

Olive oil and healthy fats are the heart and soul of the

Mediterranean diet, providing a foundation of both health and pleasure. As you embark on your journey through the Mediterranean diet, remember that it's not just about what you eat but how you savor each bite.

Olive oil, with its rich history, culinary versatility, and numerous health benefits, exemplifies the essence of Mediterranean cuisine. It's a reminder that food is not just fuel; it's a source of joy, connection, and well-being.

In the chapters that follow, we'll continue to explore the delicious and healthful elements of the

Mediterranean diet, from the vibrant world of fruits and vegetables to the savory delights of seafood and lean proteins. Each component contributes to the unique tapestry of flavors and nutrition that make the Mediterranean diet a true masterpiece of both culinary artistry and healthy living. So, embrace the golden glow of olive oil and savor the pleasures it brings to your table and your life.

CHAPTER 7

Seafood and Lean Proteins

In the mesmerizing realm of the Mediterranean diet, seafood and lean proteins take the spotlight as a source of both nourishment and culinary delight. This chapter will navigate the azure waters of Mediterranean seafood, introduce you to the lean protein choices, and uncover the health benefits and savory flavors they bring to the table.

Seafood: A Mediterranean Treasure

The Mediterranean Sea is a culinary treasure trove, offering an abundance of seafood that has been cherished for centuries. The region's coastal communities have a deep-rooted connection to the sea, and their diets reflect this relationship. Here's why seafood is an integral part of the Mediterranean diet:

1. Nutrient-Rich: Seafood is rich in essential nutrients. It's an excellent source of high-quality protein, vitamins, and minerals. Fish, in particular, is a great source of omega-3 fatty acids, which are known for their heart-healthy benefits.

2. Omega-3 Fatty Acids: Fatty fish like salmon, mackerel, and sardines are renowned for their omega-3 content. These fatty acids are linked to reduced risk factors for heart disease, improved cognitive function, and reduced inflammation.

3. Lean Protein: Most seafood is low in saturated fat, making it a lean protein source. It's an excellent choice for those looking to maintain a healthy weight and build muscle.

**4.	Versatility**: Seafood is remarkably versatile. It can be grilled, baked, broiled, poached, or served raw in dishes like ceviche or sushi. Its delicate flavor pairs well with a variety of seasonings and ingredients.

**5.	Sustainability**: Many Mediterranean countries prioritize sustainable fishing practices, ensuring the long-term health of seafood populations. This commitment to sustainability aligns with the Mediterranean diet's focus on harmony with nature.

6. Cultural Significance: Seafood has deep cultural significance in Mediterranean regions, where fishing traditions have been passed down through generations. It's often associated with communal gatherings and celebrations.

Common Mediterranean Seafood Varieties

The Mediterranean Sea offers a diverse array of seafood, and its availability varies by region. Here are some common varieties enjoyed throughout the Mediterranean:

1. Mediterranean Sea Bass (Loup de Mer): A prized white fish with a mild, delicate flavor. It's often grilled whole with simple seasonings.

2. Sardines: These small, oily fish are a rich source of omega-3s. They're often grilled or marinated and are a staple in Portuguese and Spanish cuisines.

3. Mussels and Clams: These shellfish are used in a variety of dishes, from pasta to soups. They provide lean protein and are a good source of iron.

4. Calamari: Tender rings of squid are a popular appetizer or main course. They can be fried, grilled, or sautéed with herbs and garlic.

5. Anchovies: These small, flavorful fish are used to add depth of flavor to sauces, dressings, and dishes like pizza and salads.

6. Tuna: Fresh tuna is often used in Mediterranean cuisine. It can be grilled, seared, or served raw in dishes like tuna tartare.

Lean Proteins Beyond Seafood

While seafood is a star in Mediterranean cuisine, lean proteins from other sources also play a significant role. Here's a look at some lean protein options:

1. Poultry: Chicken and turkey are enjoyed in moderation. They are often marinated in Mediterranean spices and herbs and grilled or roasted.

2. Legumes: Legumes, such as chickpeas, lentils, and beans, provide plant-based protein. They are used in a variety of Mediterranean dishes, including salads, soups, and stews.

3. Lean Cuts of Meat: When red meat is consumed, it's often in smaller portions and as part of a larger dish. Lean cuts like sirloin or tenderloin are preferred.

4. Dairy: Dairy products like yogurt and cheese, especially varieties like Greek yogurt and feta cheese, provide protein and are used in Mediterranean recipes.

Health Benefits of Seafood and Lean Proteins

The inclusion of seafood and lean proteins in the Mediterranean diet offers a wide range of health benefits:

1. Heart Health: The omega-3 fatty acids found in fatty fish are associated with reduced risk factors for heart disease, including lower cholesterol levels and improved blood vessel function.

2. Weight Management: Seafood and lean proteins are excellent sources of high-quality protein, which helps promote feelings of fullness and aids in weight management.

3. Muscle Health: Protein is essential for building and maintaining muscle mass, making seafood and lean proteins valuable for overall health and physical fitness.

4. Nutrient Density: Seafood and lean proteins are nutrient-dense, providing essential vitamins and minerals, including B vitamins, iron, and zinc.

5. Balanced Diet: Including a variety of protein sources, including seafood and lean proteins, helps create a balanced and satisfying diet.

Sustainable Seafood Choices

As you explore seafood in the Mediterranean diet, it's essential to consider sustainability.

Overfishing and unsustainable fishing practices can harm marine ecosystems and threaten seafood populations. Here are some tips for making sustainable seafood choices:

1. Know Your Sources: Seek out seafood that is sourced responsibly. Look for labels like MSC (Marine Stewardship Council) or ASC (Aquaculture Stewardship Council) when shopping for seafood.

2. Choose Local: Buying locally sourced seafood can help support sustainable fishing practices and reduce the carbon footprint associated with long-distance transportation.

3. Diversify: Explore a variety of seafood options to reduce pressure on overfished species. Ask your seafood provider for information about sustainable choices in your area.

Customizing Your Protein Intake

The Mediterranean diet offers flexibility when it comes to protein sources, allowing you to customize your meals to your dietary preferences and needs:

Vegetarian and Vegan Diets: For vegetarians and vegans, the Mediterranean diet offers an array of plant-based protein sources, including legumes, nuts, seeds, and plant-based dairy alternatives.

Balanced Approach: Most individuals benefit from a balanced approach that includes a variety of protein sources, including seafood, lean meats, and plant-based options. This provides a diverse range of nutrients and flavors.

Low-Meat or Meatless Days: You can incorporate "meatless" or "low-meat" days into your

Mediterranean diet to reduce your meat consumption while still enjoying the culinary richness of seafood and plant-based proteins.

In Conclusion

Seafood and lean proteins are the dynamic duo of the Mediterranean diet, offering a wealth of health benefits and culinary pleasures. As you journey through the Mediterranean way of eating, remember that food is not just sustenance; it's a celebration of life, a connection to nature, and an opportunity to savor the flavors of tradition.

The Mediterranean Sea, with its bountiful seafood, has provided sustenance and inspiration to countless generations. Lean proteins from various sources add depth and diversity to Mediterranean meals, allowing for a rich tapestry of flavors and textures.

In the chapters that follow, we'll continue our exploration of the Mediterranean diet, from the heart-healthy fats of olive oil to the vibrant world of fruits and vegetables. Each component adds to the intricate mosaic of flavors and nutrition that make this diet a true embodiment of health and culinary pleasure. So, let the bounty of the sea and the goodness of lean proteins be your guide as you savor the timeless treasures of the Mediterranean diet.

CHAPTER 8

Herbs, Spices, and Flavorful Additions

In the captivating world of the Mediterranean diet, herbs, spices, and flavorful additions are the magic that transforms simple ingredients into culinary masterpieces. This chapter invites you to step into the aromatic gardens of the Mediterranean and discover the enchanting realm of seasonings, condiments, and other enhancements that elevate the

Mediterranean diet to a symphony of flavors.

Herbs and Spices: The Soul of Mediterranean Cuisine

Herbs and spices are the soul of Mediterranean cooking. They provide the essential flavors, aromas, and textures that make Mediterranean dishes memorable. Here's why herbs and spices hold such a special place in this culinary tradition:

1. Flavor Enrichment: Herbs and spices add depth, complexity, and nuance to dishes, turning the ordinary into the extraordinary.

They are the secret behind the Mediterranean diet's deliciousness.

2. Aromas and Bouquets: The Mediterranean region is a haven for aromatic herbs like basil, oregano, rosemary, and thyme. These herbs infuse dishes with delightful fragrances that tantalize the senses.

3. Natural Health Benefits: Many herbs and spices offer health benefits beyond their culinary appeal. They are often used for their medicinal properties, aiding digestion, reducing inflammation, and providing antioxidants.

4. Versatility: Herbs and spices are incredibly versatile. They can be used fresh or dried, whole or ground, and in both savory and sweet dishes.

5. Tradition and Culture: The use of herbs and spices in Mediterranean cuisine is deeply rooted in tradition and culture. Each region has its own unique blend of seasonings, adding character to local dishes.

Common Mediterranean Herbs and Spices

The Mediterranean region boasts a rich tapestry of herbs and spices, each contributing to the vibrant mosaic of flavors. Here are some common ones you'll encounter:

1. **Basil**: A fragrant herb with a sweet, slightly peppery flavor. It's a key ingredient in dishes like pesto and Caprese salad.

2. **Oregano**: A staple herb in Mediterranean cooking, oregano adds a robust, earthy flavor to dishes like pizza, roasted vegetables, and grilled meats.

3. **Rosemary**: Known for its piney aroma, rosemary is often used with roasted meats, potatoes,

and bread. It imparts a savory, aromatic quality.

4. Thyme: Thyme has a subtle, earthy flavor with hints of lemon and mint. It pairs beautifully with poultry, fish, and vegetables.

5. Cinnamon: While not native to the Mediterranean, cinnamon is used in some Mediterranean desserts and sweet dishes, adding warmth and sweetness.

6. Garlic: Garlic is a kitchen workhorse, used generously in Mediterranean cuisine. Its pungent flavor is a foundation for countless dishes.

7. Cumin: This spice adds a warm, earthy flavor with a hint of citrus. It's often used in Middle Eastern dishes and spice blends.

8. Paprika: Paprika comes in various varieties, from sweet to smoked. It's a staple in Mediterranean dishes like Spanish paella and Hungarian goulash.

9. Mint: Mint adds a refreshing, cool note to both savory and sweet dishes. It's commonly used in Mediterranean salads, teas, and desserts.

10. Parsley: This versatile herb is used as a garnish and to add freshness to dishes like tabbouleh and gremolata.

Enhancing Flavorful Additions

In addition to herbs and spices, the Mediterranean diet incorporates a variety of flavorful additions that elevate dishes. These ingredients enhance both the taste and nutrition of Mediterranean meals:

1. **Citrus**: Lemons, oranges, and limes are used for their zesty, tangy flavor. Citrus juices and zest brighten up marinades, dressings, and desserts.

2. Vinegars: Balsamic vinegar, red wine vinegar, and white wine vinegar are often used to add acidity and complexity to Mediterranean dishes.

3. Nuts: Almonds, walnuts, and pine nuts provide crunch, texture, and a rich, nutty flavor to salads, sauces, and desserts.

4. Olives: Olives are a quintessential Mediterranean ingredient, used in various dishes, from salads to tapenades.

5. Capers: These tiny, briny buds add a burst of flavor to dishes like chicken piccata and pasta puttanesca.

6. Dried Fruits: Dried fruits like raisins, figs, and apricots offer a natural sweetness and chewy texture to savory dishes and desserts.

7. Honey: A touch of honey adds sweetness and depth to dressings, marinades, and desserts.

8. Yogurt: Greek yogurt is a creamy, tangy addition to both sweet and savory Mediterranean dishes.

Health Benefits of Herbs, Spices, and Flavorful Additions

The inclusion of herbs, spices, and flavorful additions in the Mediterranean diet offers more than just a feast for the senses. Here's a glimpse into the health benefits they provide:

1. Antioxidants: Many herbs and spices are rich in antioxidants, which help protect cells from oxidative damage and inflammation.

2. Anti-Inflammatory Effects: Certain spices, like turmeric, are known for their potent anti-inflammatory properties, which may help reduce the risk of chronic diseases.

3. Digestive Aid: Some herbs and spices aid digestion by promoting healthy gut function and reducing digestive discomfort.

4. Flavor Enhancement: The use of herbs, spices, and flavorful additions allows for reduced salt and sugar intake while maintaining the deliciousness of dishes.

5. Culinary Creativity: These ingredients provide endless opportunities for culinary creativity, making it easier to enjoy a varied and balanced diet.

Customizing Flavors to Your Taste

One of the joys of the Mediterranean diet is its adaptability to personal preferences. Here are some ways to customize flavors to your liking:

1. **Heat Levels**: Adjust the level of heat in your dishes by choosing mild or spicy varieties of spices like paprika or chili flakes.

2. **Herb Combinations**: Experiment with different herb

combinations to create unique flavor profiles for your dishes.

3. Seasonal Choices: Use herbs and spices that are in season for the freshest and most vibrant flavors.

4. Condiments: Explore Mediterranean condiments like harissa, tahini, and tzatziki to add depth to your dishes.

5. Personalize: Tailor the use of herbs and spices to your taste buds. Some individuals prefer more pungent flavors, while others enjoy milder seasonings.

In Conclusion

Herbs, spices, and flavorful additions are the artistic palette of the Mediterranean diet, allowing you to paint a world of flavors and aromas. As you embrace these seasonings and enhancements in your culinary journey, remember that the Mediterranean way of eating is not just about nourishing your body but also celebrating the art of flavor.

In the chapters that follow, we'll continue to unravel the Mediterranean diet, from the succulent proteins of seafood and lean meats to the vibrant world of fruits and vegetables. Each component adds to the symphony of flavors and nutrition that make the Mediterranean diet a true masterpiece of both taste and health. So, let the aromatic embrace of herbs, spices, and flavorful additions be your guide as you savor the enchanting heritage of Mediterranean cuisine.

CHAPTER 9

Fruits and Vegetables: Nature's Bounty

In the captivating landscape of the Mediterranean diet, fruits and vegetables take center stage as the jewels of nature's bounty. This chapter invites you to stroll through sun-kissed orchards and lush gardens, exploring the vibrant world of produce that defines the essence of Mediterranean cuisine. Here, we'll uncover why fruits and vegetables are the heart of this dietary tradition, the health benefits they offer, and how to make them the star of your meals.

Fruits and Vegetables: The Essence of Mediterranean Cuisine

Fruits and vegetables are the essence of Mediterranean cuisine, revered for their abundance, freshness, and colorful variety. Their significance in this diet can be understood through these key points:

1. **Abundance and Seasonality**: The Mediterranean region boasts a favorable climate that supports the year-round

cultivation of fruits and vegetables. Their availability varies with the seasons, emphasizing the importance of eating seasonally.

2. Diversity: The Mediterranean diet celebrates diversity in produce. From crisp apples and juicy tomatoes to sweet figs and tender artichokes, there's a kaleidoscope of flavors and textures to enjoy.

3. Freshness and Simplicity: Mediterranean cuisine places a premium on freshness and simplicity. Many dishes feature raw or minimally processed fruits and vegetables to showcase their natural flavors.

4. Fiber and Nutrients: Fruits and vegetables are rich in dietary fiber, vitamins, minerals, and antioxidants. They provide essential nutrients while promoting digestive health and overall well-being.

5. Culinary Versatility: Whether as the star of a salad, the foundation of a sauce, or the sweet ending to a meal, fruits and vegetables are incredibly versatile in Mediterranean cooking.

Common Mediterranean Fruits and Vegetables

The Mediterranean region is home to an extensive array of fruits and vegetables, each offering its unique contribution to the Mediterranean diet. Here are some common ones:

Fruits:

1. **Tomatoes**: A Mediterranean staple, these are used in everything from salads to sauces like marinara and gazpacho.
2. **Olives**: While technically a fruit, olives are often treated

as vegetables in culinary applications. They're integral to Mediterranean cuisine, appearing in dishes, snacks, and olive oils.

3. **Citrus Fruits**: Lemons, oranges, and grapefruits lend their tangy, aromatic flavors to marinades, dressings, and desserts.

4. **Figs**: Sweet and succulent, figs are enjoyed fresh or dried. They're used in both sweet and savory dishes.

5. **Grapes**: Grapes are a Mediterranean classic, enjoyed fresh, dried as raisins, or pressed into wine.

6. **Pomegranates**:
Pomegranate seeds add a
burst of color and flavor to
salads and desserts.

Vegetables:

1. **Eggplant**: Used in dishes
like moussaka and baba
ghanoush, eggplant is prized
for its creamy texture and
mild flavor.

2. **Zucchini**: Zucchini is a
versatile vegetable, used in
dishes like ratatouille and
stuffed zucchini flowers.

3. **Bell Peppers**: These
colorful vegetables are used

in salads, sauces, and roasted dishes.

4. **Artichokes**: Artichokes are a Mediterranean delicacy, often enjoyed in pasta dishes or simply steamed with olive oil and herbs.

5. **Spinach**: This leafy green is a common addition to Mediterranean salads, pies, and sautéed dishes.

6. **Cucumbers**: Cucumbers are refreshing and frequently used in salads, tzatziki, and chilled soups.

Health Benefits of Fruits and Vegetables

The Mediterranean diet's emphasis on fruits and vegetables contributes significantly to its numerous health benefits. Here's a glimpse into how these natural treasures support well-being:

1. Nutrient Density: Fruits and vegetables are nutrient-dense, providing essential vitamins, minerals, and antioxidants with relatively few calories.

2. Heart Health: The fiber, potassium, and antioxidants in fruits and vegetables help support heart health by reducing blood pressure and cholesterol levels.

3. Weight Management: Their high fiber content promotes feelings of fullness, aiding in weight management by reducing overall calorie intake.

4. Digestive Health: The dietary fiber in these foods supports healthy digestion, regular bowel movements, and a balanced gut microbiome.

5. Antioxidants: Fruits and vegetables are rich in antioxidants, which help protect cells from oxidative damage and reduce the risk of chronic diseases.

6. Reduced Inflammation: Certain fruits and vegetables, like berries and leafy greens, are known for their anti-inflammatory properties, which can help reduce the risk of inflammatory conditions.

7. Skin Health: The vitamins and antioxidants in these foods contribute to healthy, glowing skin by protecting it from damage and aging.

Incorporating Fruits and Vegetables Into Your Diet

Making fruits and vegetables a focal point of your Mediterranean-inspired meals is both nutritious and flavorful. Here are some tips for incorporating them into your diet:

1. Colorful Plates: Aim to fill your plate with a variety of colorful fruits and vegetables. Different colors often indicate different nutrient profiles, so a colorful plate is a well-rounded one.

2. Fresh and Seasonal: Opt for fresh, seasonal produce when possible. In-season fruits and vegetables are often at their peak in flavor and nutritional value.

3. Snack Smart: Keep fresh fruits and vegetable snacks readily available for convenient and healthy between-meal munching.

4. Salads: Create vibrant salads by combining leafy greens with an assortment of colorful vegetables, fruits, nuts, and a simple olive oil-based dressing.

5. Smoothies: Blend fruits and vegetables into smoothies for a nutritious and portable meal or snack.

6. Sides and Accompaniments: Serve fruits and vegetables as sides or accompaniments to main dishes, enhancing the overall flavor and nutrition of your meal.

7. Roasting and Grilling: Roasting and grilling vegetables can bring out their natural sweetness and create delightful caramelization.

Customizing for Dietary Preferences

The Mediterranean diet's emphasis on fruits and vegetables makes it adaptable to various dietary preferences:

Vegetarian and Vegan Diets: For vegetarians and vegans, fruits and vegetables are the cornerstones of a Mediterranean-inspired plant-based diet.

Balanced Approach: Most individuals benefit from a balanced approach that includes a variety of fruits and vegetables along with other components of the Mediterranean diet.

Low-Carb Diets: While the Mediterranean diet is not inherently low-carb, you can customize it by focusing on lower-carb fruits and vegetables like leafy greens, peppers, and berries.

In Conclusion

Fruits and vegetables are the crown jewels of the Mediterranean diet, offering a symphony of colors, flavors, and nutrients. As you explore these natural treasures in your culinary journey, remember that the Mediterranean way of eating is not just about nourishing your body but also celebrating the gifts of nature.

In the chapters that follow, we'll continue our exploration of the Mediterranean diet, from the heart-healthy fats of olive oil to the succulent proteins of seafood and lean meats. Each component adds to the rich tapestry of flavors and nutrition that make the Mediterranean diet a true embodiment of health and culinary pleasure. So, let the vibrant bounty of fruits and vegetables be your guide as you savor the timeless gifts of Mediterranean cuisine.

CHAPTER 10

The Mediterranean Diet in Practice: Meal Planning and Tips

In this final chapter of our journey through the Mediterranean diet, we'll bring all the elements together and explore practical ways to embrace this nourishing and delicious way of eating. From meal planning to culinary tips, we'll provide guidance to help you effortlessly incorporate the Mediterranean diet into your lifestyle.

Meal Planning: Creating Mediterranean-Inspired Menus

Meal planning is a cornerstone of the Mediterranean diet. It helps ensure that you enjoy a balanced and varied diet while making the most of seasonal ingredients. Here are some steps to create Mediterranean-inspired menus:

1. Embrace Seasonality: Start by choosing fruits and vegetables that are in season. They are not only fresher but also more affordable.

2. Balance Your Plate: Mediterranean meals are characterized by a balance of fruits, vegetables, lean proteins, whole grains, and healthy fats. Aim to include a variety of these components in each meal.

3. Colorful Plates: Think in terms of colors. A plate full of vibrant colors often indicates a well-balanced and nutritious meal. Aim to have at least three different colors on your plate.

4. Whole Grains: Choose whole grains like whole wheat, barley, and quinoa over refined grains.

They are higher in fiber and nutrients.

5. Plant-Based Proteins: Incorporate plant-based proteins like legumes (beans, lentils), nuts, and seeds into your meals. They add protein and variety to your diet.

6. Healthy Fats: Use extra virgin olive oil as your primary cooking fat and for dressings. You can also include fatty fish, nuts, and seeds as sources of healthy fats.

7. Portion Control: Pay attention to portion sizes. Mediterranean meals often feature smaller portions of meat and larger portions of fruits, vegetables, and whole grains.

8. Flavor with Herbs and Spices: Experiment with Mediterranean herbs and spices to enhance the flavor of your dishes while reducing the need for salt.

Sample Mediterranean Menus

To help you get started with meal planning, here are some sample Mediterranean-inspired menus for a day:

Breakfast:

- Greek yogurt topped with honey, walnuts, and fresh berries.
- Whole-grain toast with avocado, tomato, and a sprinkle of feta cheese.

Lunch:

- Greek salad with tomatoes, cucumbers, red onion, olives, and feta cheese. Drizzle with olive oil and balsamic vinegar.
- Hummus and vegetable wrap using whole-grain flatbread.

Snack:

- Fresh fruit salad with a squeeze of lemon juice and a sprinkle of cinnamon.

Dinner:

- Grilled or baked salmon with a lemon and herb marinade.
- Quinoa pilaf with sautéed spinach and garlic.
- Steamed broccoli with a drizzle of olive oil and a sprinkle of pine nuts.

Culinary Tips for Mediterranean Cooking

Here are some culinary tips to enhance your Mediterranean cooking experience:

1. Fresh Ingredients: Prioritize fresh, high-quality ingredients. The quality of your ingredients greatly influences the final flavor of your dishes.

2. Olive Oil: Invest in a good-quality extra virgin olive oil. It's not just a cooking ingredient but also a flavor enhancer.

3. Season Liberally: Don't be shy with Mediterranean herbs and spices. They are key to creating authentic flavors.

4. Slow Cooking: Some Mediterranean dishes, like stews and braises, benefit from slow cooking. It allows flavors to meld and intensify.

5. Sauces and Dips: Experiment with Mediterranean sauces and dips like tzatziki, tahini, and pesto. They can transform simple dishes into culinary delights.

6. Use Citrus: Citrus fruits like lemons and oranges add brightness to dishes. A squeeze of lemon juice can be a game-changer.

7. Be Mindful of Salt: Use salt sparingly. The Mediterranean diet is generally low in added salt, relying on herbs and spices for flavor.

8. Try New Ingredients: Don't be afraid to explore new ingredients like artichokes, capers, and different types of olives. They can add excitement to your dishes.

9. Family Style: Mediterranean meals are often served family-style, encouraging communal dining and conversation.

10. Savor the Moment: Embrace the Mediterranean philosophy of enjoying meals slowly, savoring each bite, and relishing the company of loved ones.

Customizing the Mediterranean Diet to Your Lifestyle

The Mediterranean diet is adaptable to various lifestyles and dietary preferences:

Vegetarian and Vegan: Vegetarians and vegans can easily embrace the Mediterranean diet by focusing on plant-based proteins, legumes, nuts, seeds, and plenty of fruits and vegetables.

Gluten-Free: Many Mediterranean dishes are

naturally gluten-free. Opt for gluten-free grains like quinoa, rice, and cornmeal, and check labels for hidden gluten in sauces and processed foods.

Low-Carb: To lower the carbohydrate content, focus on non-starchy vegetables, lean proteins, and healthy fats. Limit grains and opt for whole grains when you do include them.

Dairy-Free: Substitute dairy products with dairy-free alternatives like almond milk, coconut yogurt, or vegan cheese if you have dairy restrictions.

Low-Sodium: If you need to reduce sodium intake, use herbs, spices, and citrus to flavor your dishes instead of salt. Avoid processed foods, which often contain high levels of sodium.

In Conclusion

The Mediterranean diet is not just a way of eating; it's a way of living, celebrating the pleasures of food, and embracing a balanced, healthy lifestyle. As you embark on your Mediterranean journey, remember that it's not about perfection but about making gradual, sustainable changes that suit your taste and preferences.

From the sun-drenched orchards of fruits to the aromatic gardens of herbs and spices, each component of the Mediterranean diet contributes to a tapestry of flavors and nutrition that is both satisfying and nourishing. With meal planning, culinary tips, and customization options, you can make this timeless and delicious way of eating a part of your daily life.

As you continue your culinary adventure beyond this guide, may the Mediterranean diet be a source of joy, health, and connection, inviting you to savor the timeless traditions and natural wonders of Mediterranean cuisine.

CONCLUSION

In the pages of this book, we've embarked on a flavorful journey through the captivating world of the Mediterranean diet, a culinary tradition that is as nourishing as it is delicious. From the sun-soaked landscapes of olive groves to the azure waters teeming with seafood treasures, we've explored the rich tapestry of flavors, ingredients, and health benefits that define this way of eating.

The Mediterranean diet isn't just a diet; it's a celebration of life, a communion with nature, and a testament to the joys of food. It's a philosophy that encourages us to savor each bite, to cherish the simple pleasures of a shared meal, and to embrace the wisdom of generations past who understood the profound connection between what we eat and how we live.

As we conclude this culinary odyssey, let us remember the key lessons we've uncovered:

1. A Symphony of Flavors: The Mediterranean diet is a symphony of flavors, where each ingredient plays its unique note, contributing to a harmonious and memorable dining experience.

2. Health and Well-being: Beyond its delectable taste, the Mediterranean diet offers a wealth of health benefits, from heart health to reduced inflammation and a lower risk of chronic diseases.

3. Flexibility and Adaptability: This way of eating is flexible, accommodating various dietary preferences and needs, from vegetarian to low-carb to gluten-free.

4. Seasonal and Sustainable: It encourages us to eat seasonally and sustainably, forging a deeper connection with the natural world and supporting responsible food production.

5. Simplicity and Pleasure: It reminds us that the simple act of sharing a meal with loved ones, savoring each bite, and delighting in the art of flavor is a source of immense pleasure and well-being.

6. A Way of Life: The Mediterranean diet is not a quick-fix solution; it's a way of life. It invites us to make gradual, sustainable changes that lead to lasting health and happiness.

As you journey forward, may the Mediterranean diet be your guide, inviting you to explore new flavors, nourish your body, and celebrate the timeless traditions of Mediterranean cuisine. Whether you're preparing a family feast or sharing a simple meal with friends, may you find joy in the kitchen, connect with the beauty of nature, and savor the pleasures of good food.

In the end, the Mediterranean diet is not just about what's on your plate; it's about the life you lead around it, the moments you create, and the memories you cherish. So, here's to a life well-lived, where each meal is a reminder of the abundance and beauty that surrounds us, and each bite is a celebration of the artistry of food and the richness of life itself. Cheers to the Mediterranean diet—a journey of taste, health, and heart.

www.ingramcontent.com/pod-product-compliance
Lightning Source LLC
Chambersburg PA
CBHW050727260726
48661CB00001B/105